Pharmacy Technician Certified Board Comprehensive Pharmacy Math

Anne Yen Nguyen

Copyright © 2019 by Anne Yen Nguyen.

Library of Congress Control Number:		2019908594
ISBN:	Hardcover	978-1-7960-4325-9
	Softcover	978-1-7960-4326-6
	eBook	978-1-7960-4324-2

All rights reserved. No part of this book may be reproduced or transmitted in any form or by any means, electronic or mechanical, including photocopying, recording, or by any information storage and retrieval system, without permission in writing from the copyright owner.

The authors and the publisher make no warranties of any kind and shall not be held liable for any special, consequential, or other damages that result in whole or in part from the reader's use of or reliance on this material. By following the guidelines and instructions contained in this material, the reader willingly assumes all risks incurred in connection with such instructions. Further, none of the products or services described in this manual are warranted or guaranteed by the author or the publisher.

Any people depicted in stock imagery provided by Getty Images are models, and such images are being used for illustrative purposes only.
Certain stock imagery © Getty Images.

Print information available on the last page.

Rev. date: 08/08/2019

To order additional copies of this book, contact:
Xlibris
1-888-795-4274
www.Xlibris.com
Orders@Xlibris.com

Contents

Acknowledgments 5
Preface 7
Chapter 1. Pharmacy Introduction 9
Chapter 2. Pharmacy Technicians' Duties 11
Chapter 3. Basic Mathematics Review 14
Chapter 4. Pharmacy Conversion Systems 26
Chapter 5. Temperature Conversions 30
Chapter 6. Roman Numeral System 33
Chapter 7. Drug Enforcement Agency Determination 36
Chapter 8. Fractions and Decimals 38
Chapter 9. Ratio and Proportion 41
Chapter 10. Milliequivalents and Milliosmoles 44
Chapter 11. Percentage, Percentage Strength, and Ratio Strength 49
Chapter 12. Calculating Dosage 53
Chapter 13. Calculating Day Supply 58
Chapter 14. Calculating Children's Dosage 62
Chapter 15. Dilution Method 64
Chapter 16. Pharmacy Alligations 68
Chapter 17. Flow Rate Calculation 73
Chapter 18. Commercial Calculations and Terminology 76
Appendix A. Patterned Plan of Attack for Questions 79
Appendix B. Patterned Plan of Attack for Calculations 81
Appendix C. Common Pharmacy Abbreviations 85
Appendix D. Common Medical Abbreviations 87
Answers 93
References 97
Index 99

Acknowledgments

To our families, the time that they have sacrificed so that this edition will become a reality.

To our mentors and advisors, whose vision provided education and motivation that encouraged our professional growth and challenged us to be innovators in our educational endeavors.

To my family, peers, and students who have shared their thoughts regarding the content and format of this text.

In memory of my father, your impact and contribution to my life is the greatest gift I could receive. I would not be enjoying the success and life I have today without your love and support; as well as the courage and vision you had in helping our family escape the communist regime in Vietnam to come to America, so that we would have the opportunity to grow and pursue our own dreams in a free and democratic country.

Preface

This textbook is intended to assist students who wish to become pharmacy technicians, with or without any pharmacy-related experience. To be a pharmacy technician, one needs to be proficient in math. It is necessary in order to accurately mix medications, measure fluids, calculate drug dosages, day supply, pricing, and so forth. Careers in the pharmaceutical industry are consistently in high demand. Becoming a nationally certified pharmacy technician is not that difficult. One would need to pass the National Certified Pharmacy Board exam with a 70 percent in the following areas:

1. Assisting the pharmacist in serving patients
2. Maintaining medication and inventory control systems
3. Participating in the administration and management of pharmacy practice

This book is designed for any student wanting to strengthen their abilities in pharmacy math to pass the National Certified Pharmacy Board exam. Passing the exam depends on the student's time spent in study. This book has eighteen short chapters, which covers all different areas of pharmacy math. The Pharmacy Technician Certified Board Comprehensive Pharmacy Math book provides for all the possible pharmacy math questions anticipated on the technician board exam.

Many students who have purchased this book, along with our other textbooks, and have study diligently have passed with a high score. This textbook is provided by the PTCB preparation team for interested individuals pursuing a rewarding career as a certified pharmacy technician.

Chapter 1

Pharmacy Introduction

Pharmacy technicians today play an important role in the pharmacy business in hospital, retail and other pharmacy settings. Technicians interact with nurses, pharmacists, and health insurance providers. They work under the pharmacist's supervision and are allowed to assist in pharmacy activities that do not require the professional judgment of a pharmacist. Technicians are becoming more involved in the production and technical aspects of pharmacy, while pharmacists have become more involved with patient-care activities and are the dispensers of medicine.

Pharmacy technicians assist registered pharmacists in filling and dispensing prescriptions and other technician tasks. As pharmacy technicians, they will use their math skills on a daily basis. However, basic math can be easily forgotten when it is not used routinely. This book will help one review the fundamentals of calculations and how those calculations are applied within the pharmacy.

Certified Pharmacy Technician (CPhT) is a title given to individuals who have passed the national PTCB exam and have a current, valid PTCB certificate. This title implies that an individual has had additional training, which will make them more marketable and valuable in the pharmaceutical industry. In order to be a pharmacy technician, one must be highly skilled in basic math; such as addition, subtraction, multiplication, division, roman numerals, and fractions. On a daily basis, the technician will use these skills for tasks such as dosage and day supply calculations, counting pills, finalizing customer invoices, and interpreting prescriptions that are written in roman numerals.

Thus, these fundamental pharmacy math concepts are foundations for the more complicated and advanced skills needed in the pharmacy business. Thorough knowledge of pharmacy math is highly beneficial to anyone working in the pharmacy industry. An understanding of business math would also be essential for maintaining product inventory and calculating markups and discounts.

Chapter 2

Pharmacy Technicians' Duties

Focus on the Patient

1. Enter prescription order into the computer.
    a. Receive medication order from the patient's chart or prescription via fax, telephone, electronic prescribing, or directly from the patient.
2. Collect data from patient (name, date of birth, address, insurance).
3. Maintain patient medication profile (drug allergies or other medications/herbals).
4. Help pharmacists with education programs about diseases, devices, and durable medical equipment (DME).
5. Call physicians' offices for refill requests (done in retail pharmacy).
    a. This is a courtesy procedure for patients.
6. Document authorization for refill approvals (by fax, phone, or computer).
7. Help patients find over-the-counter (OTC) products.

Dispense Functions

1. Accurately prepare IV (intravenous) solutions with approved training done in hospitals.
2. Make bulk supplies (bulk compounding). This is usually seen in retail or community pharmacy.
3. Compound prescriptions with training.
    Compounding is the preparation of sterile, nonsterile, cytotoxic, and hazardous products for a specific patient.
4. Perform calculations for medication order or compound using measured amounts.
5. Reconstitute solid preparations into liquids or suspensions.

Example: Amoxil 250 mg / 5 mL reconstituted with distilled water
6. Count and pour medications into prescription vials or bottles.
7. Include labels and auxiliary labels on vials or bottles.
8. Handle hazardous wastes properly.
9. Bill third party (health insurances) for services and medications.
10. File prescriptions according to laws and regulations.
    a. Controlled and noncontrolled prescriptions are usually kept separately.
        i. Three separate files
            - One file for Schedule II prescriptions
            - One file for Schedule III to V prescriptions
            - One file for all noncontrolled prescriptions
    b. Keep files for several years, depending on the requirement of the state's board of pharmacy. Federal requirements are to keep all prescriptions records according to the state law.
11. Help keep accurate records for the pharmacy department.
12. Perform basic calculations associated with the business aspect of pharmacy.

Inventory Control

1. Assist in inventory control.
2. Purchase drugs, OTCs, and accessories.
3. Check in order to verify all packages on the invoices should be matched with you have received.
4. Separate invoices from controlled and noncontrolled medications and file it away. It should readily retrievable upon inspection.
5. Maintain inventory on shelf.
6. Maintain controlled substance inventory (narcotics etc.).
7. Process returns for credit into inventory.
    a. Send back expired drugs, overstocked drugs, or recalled drugs to manufacturers.

8. Keep pharmacy department supplies well stocked.

To answer questions about technician duties, use *common sense*. The pharmacy technician can handle questions and answer phone calls that do not require a pharmacist's judgment. Being part of a pharmacy team, it's important for technicians to adhere the pharmacy's policies and procedures, as well as the pharmacist's instructions precisely. Everything the technician and staff do shapes the image of the pharmacy.

In pharmacy, we usually use a calculator to perform our calculations for double-checking prior to giving the data to the pharmacist as a final check to help us to avoid mathematical errors.

Tasks which pharmacy technicians may *not* perform include the following:

1. Provide drug information to the patient or the patient's caregiver (patient counseling).
2. Transfer prescriptions between pharmacies.
3. Interpret patient profiles and performing drug use reviews (OBRA counseling).
4. Receive oral prescription orders by phone.
5. Interpreting and evaluating prescription drug orders.
6. Select drug products (branded versus generic). They must ask the pharmacist for state law restrictions.
7. Perform the final check of dispensed product before delivery to the patient.

These tasks are only performed by a licensed pharmacist. Remember, the pharmacist is liable for everything the technicians do or anything that happens in the pharmacy. Mistakes can seriously affect patients. You should view patients as you would your loved ones, as someone who should receive our best efforts. Thus, avoid mistakes at any cost. The healthcare field is required to be 100 percent accurate at all times.

Chapter 3

Basic Mathematics Review

I. *Addition* is a method of math that involves adding one number to another number, the result of which is the sum of the two numbers.

   a. When adding the whole integer, it is not necessary to find the lowest common denominator (LCD). You just need to add all the numbers together, and its sum will be the result of the two numbers.

   Example: $123 + 456 = 579$

   b. When adding decimals, it is not necessary to find the LCD. However, it is important to make sure that you line up the decimals in a straight line. You must use the calculator and enter the number exactly as you see the decimal.

   Example: $123.5 + 456.2 = 579.7$

   c. When adding fractions, it is very important to find the common denominator before you begin any calculation. The only time you need to find the common denominator is when you are working with adding and subtracting fractions.

   Example: $\frac{1}{4} + \frac{2}{3} + \frac{1}{2} =$

   Find the lowest common denominator. Think of the least common multiple of the denominators (4, 3, 2), which for this instance would be 12.

Another method is that you can multiply all the denominators together. In this case, let's multiply: 4 × 3 × 2 = 24. Then simplify to 12.

If the bottom number (also known as the denominator) is multiplied by 3 or 4 or 6, then do the same with your top number (also known as the numerator) by that same number. Then add the sum of all numerators together (3 + 8 + 6) = 17, and the denominator will be the same, which is the lowest common denominator 12. Thus, your answer should be $^{17}/_{12}$

$$\frac{1}{4} + \frac{2}{3} + \frac{1}{2} = \frac{1 (\times 3)}{4 (\times 3)} + \frac{2 (\times 4)}{3 (\times 4)} + \frac{1 (\times 6)}{2 (\times 6)} = \frac{3 + 8 + 6}{12} = \frac{17}{12}$$

Practice the following problems and show your work:

1. 57 + 14 =

2. 103 + 11 =

3. 453 + 319 =

4. 33 ¾ + 1,007 =

5. 3,891 + 101.59

6. (981 + 17 ¼) + 0.756

7. ($^{10}/_6$ + 1 $^{4}/_6$) + 1.589

8. (239.51 + 0.964) + 384 ¼

9. (11,389 ⅕ + 68 $^{5}/_9$) + 8,974.46

10. (569,478 + 7,216 $^{8}/_9$) + 2,576.8957

II. *Subtraction* is a method of math that involves subtracting one number from another number. A smaller number is usually subtracted from a larger number, and the result will be the difference of the two.

    a. *Subtracting whole numbers or integers.* The simplest method is simply taking the difference between the two numbers.

    Example: $201 - 100 = 101$

    b. *Subtracting decimals.* Keep in mind that you have to make sure that you line up your decimals before you begin your calculation.

    Example: $871.9 - 254.3 = 617.6$

    or   871.**9**
         - 254.**3**
          617.6

    c. *Subtracting fractions.* It is very important to find the common denominator before you begin your calculation.

    Example: $\frac{2}{3} - \frac{1}{4} =$

$$\frac{2\,(\times 4)}{12} \quad - \quad \frac{1(\times 3)}{12} \quad = \quad \frac{8-3}{12} \quad = \quad \frac{5}{12}$$

        a. What is the lowest common denominator of these two bottom numbers to which 3 and 4 would go? The answer is 12. You can multiply the two numbers together, and it will equal to 12.

b. If you multiply your denominators 3 by 4, you will get 12, then the numerator will also need to be multiplied by the same number—2 multiplied by 4 equals 8. Again, if my bottom number 4 multiplied by 3 is equal to 12, then my top number 1 also needs to be multiplied by 3 to get 3.

c. Then if you take the difference between 8 and 3, my answer is 5. Thus, the answer is 5/12.

Practice the following problems, and show your work:

1. $183 - 121 =$

2. $161 - 59 =$

3. $651 - 359 =$

4. $859\ 3/4 - 497\ 1/4 =$

5. $4{,}891.596 - 2{,}456.56 =$

6. $3{,}895.215 - 1{,}259.21 =$

7. $8{,}951\ 9/15 - 1{,}189\ 3/4 =$

8. $(2{,}503 - 685.78) - 213.2 =$

9. $(3{,}001 - 111.89) - 879.21 =$

10. $5{,}963\ 2/3 - 1{,}189.33 =$

III. *Multiplication* is a method of math that involves multiplying all numbers together to get the product of these numbers. The symbol × stands for multiplication. The symbol of multiplication is *, as shown on the calculator.

    a. *Multiplication of whole integers*. This is the simplest method. You just need to multiply all the numbers together.

       Example: 251 × 142 = 35,642
              or 251 * 142 = 35,642

    b. *Multiplication of decimals*. When working with this method, be sure to count all your decimals.

       1. Example: 74.**21** × 21.**6** =

         Note: This example has a total of three numbers behind the decimal.

         If you input it in your calculator, the result will be 1,602.**936**

         Answer: 74.**21** × 21.**6** = 1,602.**936**

       2. Here's another example: 71.**25** × 20.**4** =

         If you multiply 71.25 with 20.4, you will get 1,453.5. It should be 1,453.**500**. Remember, you should have a total of three numbers behind the decimal, but those zeros are understood.

         Answer: 71.25 × 20.4 = 1,453.**5**

c. *Multiplication of fractions.* Just simply multiply the top numbers and the bottom numbers together then reduce to the lowest term.
Example:

$$\frac{2}{3} \times \frac{5}{8} = \frac{2 \times 5}{3 \times 8} = \frac{10}{24} = \frac{5}{12}$$

Practice the following problems, and show your work:

1. 119 × 281 =

2. 298 × 374 =

3. 516 × 13 =

4. 159 × 1,002 =

5. 987 × 654.0 =

6. 1,523 × 759.23 =

7. 2,463 × 1,459 =

8. 2,891 × 3,524 =

9. 10,522 × 975 ½ =

10. 4,596.35 × 531 ¼ =

IV. *Division* is a method of math using the divided line. The top number is divided by the bottom number.

    a. *Division of whole numbers.* This is the opposite of multiplying whole numbers. It is the process where we try to find out how many times a number (divisor) is contained in another number (dividend).

    Example: $33 \div 11 = 3$

    b. *Division of decimal numbers.* If the divisor is not a whole number, move decimal point to the right to make it a whole number then move the decimal point in the dividend the same number of places. Divide as usual. Keep dividing until the answer terminates or repeats.

    Example: $5.0 \div 0.5 = 10$

    c. *Division of fractions.* When solving a division problem by multiplying by the reciprocal, remember to write all whole numbers and mixed numbers as improper fractions. The final answer should be simplified and written as a mixed number.

    Example: $3/8 \div 1/3$
                 $3/8 \times 3/1 = 9/8 = 1\ 1/8$

Practice the following problems:

1. $9/5 \div 1/4 =$

2. $59 \div 7 =$

3. $126 \div 12 =$

4. $436 \div 57.5 =$

5. $718 \div 64 \frac{1}{2} =$

6. $543.65 \div 13 \frac{5}{8} =$

7. $2{,}341 \div 271.125 =$

8. $611 \frac{2}{3} \div 125.75 =$

9. $(971.564 \div 120.25) \div 13 =$

10. $(1{,}001 \frac{1}{4} \div 26 \frac{3}{4}) \div 9 =$

The Metric System

mcg	mg	cg	dg	gm	dg	hg	kg	Mg
micro	milli	centi	deci	gram	deka	hecto	kilo	mega
0.000001	0.001	0.01	0.1	1	10	100	1,000	1,000,000

Please commit the above chart to memory.
This chart is very useful to determine the conversion to the metric system (meter, gram or liter). The metric measurement is based on the powers of ten.
If you convert the desired number to the right, you would need to move the decimal point three spaces right as well, you will gain three zeros.

For example: Convert 1 gram to mg.

$$1 \times 1\,000 = 1000$$

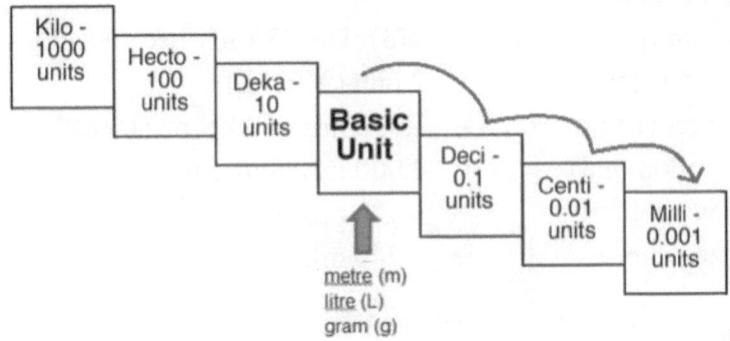

Chapter 4

Pharmacy Conversion Systems

There are two types of pharmaceutical systems: apothecary and avoirdupois. Among these systems, the metric system is well-known because of its international use among the health-care professionals.

Pharmacy technicians need to know these different systems of measurement for both liquids and solids.

Here is a list of the most common pharmaceutical conversions used in pharmacies.

Conversions are usually on the sig part of a prescription.

Volume
- 1 milliliter (mL) = 16 minim (m) (~ 20 drops [gtts])
- 1 fluid dram = 5 mL
- 1 teaspoon (tsp) = 5 mL
- 1 tablespoon (tbsp) = 15 mL
- 1 ounce (oz) = 30 mL
- 1 pint (pt) = 473 mL (~ 480 mL for calculations)
- 1 quart (qt) = 2 pint (960 mL)
- 1 liter (L) = 1,000 mL or 34 fl oz (1.1 qt)
- 1 gallon (gal) = 4,000 mL (4 quarts = 8 pt)
- 1 wine glass = ~ 120 mL
- 1 tea cup = ~ 240 mL

Weight
- 1 grain (gr) = 65 mg
- 1 gram (g) = 15 gr
- 1 ounce (oz) = 30 g (480 gr)
- 1 pound (lb) = 454 g

1 kilogram (kg) = 2.2 lb
1 inch = 2.54 cm

In order to pass the board exam, the above list needs to be memorized by the student(s). When solving conversion problems, proportion is the only type of method used. For every proportion problem, there are three known values and one unknown value. Solve for that unknown value. It is very important to know how to set up the problem.

Example: How many milligrams are in a 5 gr aspirin tablet?
  a. $\dfrac{1 \text{ gr}}{65 \text{ mg}} = \dfrac{5 \text{ gr}}{x}$
  b. Cross multiply to solve for x alone.
  c. $x = 325$ mg

I. *Volume* is the amount of space occupied by an object measured in three dimensions expressed in cubic units.

Practice the following problems:

1. How many milliliters are in 7 oz?

2. How many teaspoons are in 90 mL?

3. How many milliliters are in a half gallon?

4. How many 30 mL are in a gallon of lactulose?

5. How many 6 mL are in a 7 oz metoclopramide?

6. How many pint(s) is/are in a 5.5 qt of water?

7. How many glasses (120 mL) are in 1 ¾ gal of isopropyl alcohol?

8. How many liter(s) is/are in 2.75 gal?

9. How many drops are in 8.75 mL if 1 mL has 20 gtts?

10. How many 5 mL doses can be made out of 5 fl oz?

II. *Weight* is the amount of mass of an object or person.

1. How many 100 mL doses are in 1 g?

2. How many kilograms are in a patient who weighs 27 lb?

3. How many 10 g doses are in 100 kg?

4. How many grams are in 5 oz if 1 oz (avoir) is equal to 28 g?

5. How many ounces are in 960 gr?

6. How many pounds are in 73 kg?

7. How many milligrams are in 7 gr if 1 gr is equal to 65 mg?

8. How many grains are in 585 mg if a grain is equal to 65 mg?

9. How many milligrams of amoxicillin are given to a 10 kg child for a 0.5 mg/kg per day?

10. How many milligrams of gabapentin does a patient receive per day if the prescription indicates 600 mg TID?

Chapter 5

Temperature Conversions

Fahrenheit and Celsius are the two most common temperatures used around the world. Most people are more familiar with Fahrenheit than Celsius. Normal body temperature is measured as 98.6°F. Certain medications such as all insulin, Xalatan, NuvaRing, Humira, and liquid-mixed antibiotics are required to be stored in the refrigerator. Thus, it is very important to monitor the refrigerator daily and maintain appropriate fridge temperature between 2°C and 8°C.

Converting between temperatures is very simple. Students would need to plug the number to convert the variable (either °F or °C) into the formula.

Memorize the following formulas.

$$°F = 1.8 \times C + 32 \qquad °C = 0.5556 \, (°F - 32)$$

$$°F = \frac{(9 \times C)}{5} + 32 \qquad °C = \frac{5 \times (°F - 32)}{9}$$

Convert the following temperatures to Fahrenheit:

Example on converting 23°C to Fahrenheit:

$$°F = \frac{(9 \times C)}{5} + 32 \qquad \text{or} \qquad °F = 1.8 \times C + 32$$

$$F = 1.8 \, (23) + 32 = 73.4°F$$

1. 32°C = _____ °F

2. 25°C = _____ °F

3. 14°C = _____ °F

4. 9°C = _____ °F

5. -3°C = _____ °F

6. 46°C = _____ °F

7. 58°C = _____ °F

8. 76°C = _____ °F

9. 98.6°C = _____ °F

10. 121°C = _____ °F

Convert the following temperatures to Celsius:

1. 104°F = _____ °C

2. 92°F = _____ °C

3. 76°F = _____ °C

4. 32°F = _____ °C

5. 10°F = _____ °C

6. 56°F = _____ °C

7. 78°F = _____ °C

8. 98.6°F = _____ °C

9. 110°F = _____ °C

10. Xalatan eye drops are to be stored in a temperature between 2°C and 8°C.
   What is the correct temperature in Fahrenheit?
   a. 20.5°F and 36.4°F
   b. 25°F and 45°F
   c. 30.5°F and 40.5°F
   d. 35.6°F and 46.4°F

Chapter 6

Roman Numeral System

ss	=	½	V	=	5,000
I	=	1	X	=	10,000
V	=	5	L	=	50,000
X	=	10	C	=	100,000
L	=	50	D	=	500,000
C	=	100	M	=	1,000,000
D	=	500			
M	=	1,000			

These are the rules for interpreting roman numerals:
1. Always read from left to right.
2. Always write roman numerals from a larger value to a smaller value.
3. Never write more than three of the same symbol in a row.
4. Always *add* from right to left if a second roman numeral is a smaller value.
5. Always *subtract* from left to right if a second roman numeral is a larger value.

It is best to always group them in thousandths, hundredths, tenths, and ones.
Then find the roman numeral to match it.

Example:

a. Convert regular number to roman numeral

Eight is written as **VIII** (5 + 1 + 1 + 1).

Nine is written as **IX** (10 - 1 or 10 less than 1).

Eleven is written as **XI** (10 + 1).

Twenty-four is written as **XXIV** (10 + 10 + 4).

b. Convert roman number to regular number

124 = 100 + 20 + 4. This would be written as C + XX + IV = CXXIV.

321 = 300 + 20 + 1. This would be written as CCC + XX + I = CCCXXI.

506 = 500 + 6 = D + VI. This would be written as DVI.

1998 = 1,000 + 900 + 90 + 8 = M + CM + XC + VIII. This would be written as MCMXCVIII.

Convert the following roman numerals into arabic numbers.

1. XCIV
2. DCCLVIII
3. CDXCIII
4. MCMXCVIII
5. MCMXCI
6. MMV
7. MMXXIII
8. MMCXXXVII
9. MMMDCCLXXXV
10. MVLXXXIX

Translate the following arabic numbers into roman numerals.

1. 19
2. 34
3. 49
4. 114
5. 241
6. 579
7. 681
8. 978
9. 1,021
10. 5,369

Chapter 7

Drug Enforcement Agency Determination

Each subscriber has his/her own DEA number. This number is very important for prescribing controlled prescriptions (e.g., anxiolytics, sedatives, hypnotics, pain medications, and other narcotics). These are issued to the physician from the Drug Enforcement Administration. There is a method to validate whether this number is correct by determining the last digit of the physician DEA number and to make sure that this last digit matches the DEA number written on controlled prescriptions. The first two characters are letters, and the last seven are numbers. The first letter is always either *A*, *B*, *F*, *G*, or *M*. The second letter of the DEA number is the first letter of the physician's last name.

Here are the rules in determining the last digit of the physician's DEA number:
1. Add the first, third, and fifth digits together.
2. Add the second, fourth, and sixth digits together, then multiply this sum by two.
3. Then add these two sums together. The number on the right of the sum would be the seventh digit.

Examples on Calculating the Drug Enforcement Agency Number:

1. Add the odd numbers (first, third, and fifth): $1 + 3 + 5 = 9$.
2. Add the even numbers (second, fourth, and sixth): $2 + 4 + 6 = 12 \times 2 = 24$.
3. Add the sum of both steps together: $9 + 24 = 33$.
4. The second digit of the sum is the last digit of the DEA number.

Answer: AB 1234563

1. What is the last digit of the DEA number BD 987654?
    a. 9
    b. 8
    c. 7
    d. 6

2. Which of the following is the correct DEA number?
    a. AS 5352613
    b. AE 5555557
    c. AD 1111119
    d. BC 2387156

3. Calculate the last digit of the following DEA numbers.
    a. AB 535123_
    b. BS 781245_

Chapter 8

Fractions and Decimals

Different Types of Fractions

1. Proper fraction   ex.: ½
2. Improper fraction   ex.: 4/2
3. Complex fraction   ex.: ⅔ / ½
4. Mixed number   ex.: 3 ½

Fractions

    a. *Addition of fractions*   ex.: ½ + ¼ = x
    b. *Subtraction of fractions*   ex.: ¾ − ¼ = x

    Note: Before solving problems with adding or subtracting fractions, it is important to obtain the lowest common denominator for the two fractions.

    c. *Multiplication of fractions*   ex.: ⅝ × ⅓ = x

    Note: First, multiply the numerators of the fraction to get the new numerator. Then multiply the denominators of the fraction to get the new denominator. Be sure to reduce it to the lowest term.

    d. *Division of fractions*   ex.: ¾ ÷ ¼ = x

    Note: To divide a number by a fraction, multiply the number by the reciprocal of the fraction. Then multiply the numerators and denominators just like in basic multiplication.

Decimals

    a. *Addition and subtraction of decimals*

Note: Make sure to align the decimals points first, then add each column of digits, starting on the right and working to the left.

Example:

$$51.3 + 26.1 = 77.4$$

$$96.3 - 16.2 = 80.1$$

b. *Multiplication of decimals*

Note: First, multiply the numbers as if they were whole numbers. Then count the total decimal points and place it in the answer by counting starting from the right and moving the point the same number of places to the left.

Example: $\frac{1}{8} \times \frac{7}{8} = \frac{7}{64}$

c. *Division of decimals*

Note: First, divide the numbers as if they were whole numbers. Count the total decimal points and place it in the answer by counting starting from the right and moving the point the same number of places to the left.

Example: $3.6 \div 4 = 0.9$

Practice Questions for Fractions (Addition, Subtraction, Multiplication, and Division of Fractions)

1. $½ + ¾ =$ _____

2. $¾ + ⅚ =$ _____

3. $⅛ + 3/16 =$ _____

4. $¾ - ¼ =$ _____

5. $5/16 - ⅛ =$ _____

6. $⅝ - ¼ =$ _____

7. $¼ × ¼ =$ _____

8. $⅔ × ⅝ =$ _____

9. $⅖ ÷ ⅕ =$ _____

10. $9/3 ÷ ⅓ =$ _____

Practice Questions for Decimals

1. 423.65
   + 14.61

2. 523.23
   + 167.18

3. 0.671
   + 3.92

4. 3.20
   - 1.18

5. 30.313
   - 15.72

6. 316.18
   - 3.89

7. 5.8
   × 0.6

8. 1.29
   × 1.8

9. $35.0 ÷ 0.7$

10. $8.42 ÷ 2.0$

Chapter 9

Ratio and Proportion

This chapter is very useful for pharmacy technicians since it is essential and is utilized in most of the calculations necessary in this profession.

I. *Ratio* is an expression of the relationship between one number and another. In other words, it states the relationship between the two quantities *A* and *B*.

There are two ways to express ratio:
1. Colon
   Example: A:B :: C:D
   Example: 2:**3** :: *x*:9
   - Means (inside numbers) 2:**3** :: **x**:9
   - Extremes (outside numbers) **2**:3 :: *x*:**9**
   - Set up as a proportion or fraction
   $$\frac{2}{3} = \frac{x}{9}$$

   - When solving problems, cross multiply.
   - Multiply the extremes together (2 × 9).
   - Multiple the means together (3 × *x*)
   - Solve for *x*; in this case *x* = 6
   - Answer: X = 6

2. Fraction
   Example: A/B = C/D
   ⅔ = x/9
   Solving for X
   Cross and multiply   (2 x 9) = 3x
   Divide to solve for X alone ; 18 = 3X
   Solve for X alone = 6   X = 6
   Answer: X = 6

II. *Proportion* is an expression of the relationship of two equal ratios.

Rules for solving proportion problems are as follows:
1. Must be converted to the same unit (mg, mcg, mL, etc.).
2. Same units must be on the same line (A = A1). Both must have the same.
3. Must have three known values.
4. Solve for one unknown (x).

These are methods that will help solve unknown quantities when you are given three known terms.
a. Terms must have the same unit (mg, mL, etc.) before solving the problem.
b. Always express in two equal ratios (the product of the means = the product of the extremes).
c. Set up as fractions.
d. Solve for the unknown (x).

$$A/B = C/D$$
$$A:B = C:D$$

Example: Aspirin tablets are labeled 325 mg. How many grains of aspirin are in each tablet? (Note: 1 gr = 65 mg.)

$$1 \text{ gr} / 65 \text{ mg} = x / 325 \text{ mg}$$
$$65 \text{ mg} (x) = 1 \text{ gr} (325 \text{ mg})$$
$$x = 5 \text{ gr}$$

Solve the following problems:

1. How many teaspoons are in half a pint?

2. There are fifty tablets in a bottle. If every bottle contains the same number of tablets, how many tablets are in eight bottles?

3. If you receive a prescription for 0.25 mcg/kg of digoxin and the patient weighs 74 lb, what is the dose of digoxin for this patient?

4. If the doctor ordered 50 mg/kg of amoxicillin and the child weighs 32 lb, what is the dose for this child?

5. You received a prescription for 250 mg of Augmentin twice a day for ten days. You have 125 mg/5 mL 100 mL available of the drug. What is the dose for this prescription in milliliters?

6. You have a vial of digoxin injection that contains 500 mcg in 2 mL. What is the volume (in milliliter) needed to deliver for a dose of 0.250 mg?

7. A vial of insulin contains 100 units/mL. Dr. Schmidt wrote an order to give 35 units of the insulin Novolin 70/30 subcutaneous at bedtime. How many milliliters of insulin should be administered?

8. How many drops are there in two tablespoons if a milliliter is equal to 20 gtts?

9. Sodium bicarbonates are labeled 650 mg. How many grains of sodium bicarbonate are in each tablet?

10. The direction for mixing amoxicillin 250 mg / 5 mL states that when 80 mL of distilled water is added to the contents of the bottle, the resulting volume is 150 mL. What is the new concentration when only half of the amount of distilled water is added?

Chapter 10

Milliequivalents and Milliosmoles

What are *milliequivalents*? By definition, it is a unit of measurement related to the total number of ionic charges in a solution or a unit of measurement of the amount of chemical activity of an electrolyte as stated in *US Pharmacopeia*.

Electrolyte solutions are liquid preparations commonly prepared by hospital pharmacy technicians and used for the treatment of electrolyte disturbances, dehydration, and total parenteral nutrition.

It is abbreviated as *mEq*. It represents the amount in milligram of a solute equal to 1/1,000 of its gram as in weight.

These numbers (milliequivalent) are usually found on the bags of large-volume saline and dextrose solutions. For example, 0.9% NaCl contains 0.9 g NaCl in every 100 mL of solution or 15.4 mEq Na+ in every 100 mL of NS0.9% solution.

Example:

> An order called for 30 mEq KCl added to a 1,000 mL bag of normal saline. You have 2 mEq/mL of 100 mL bottle of KCl. How many milliliters of KCl is needed?
>
> Step 1: Use the proportion formula to set up an equation as follows:
>
> $$\frac{x \text{ mL}}{30 \text{ mEq}} = \frac{1 \text{ mL}}{2 \text{ mEq}}$$
>
> Step 2: Cross multiply.
>
> $$30 \times 1 = x \times 2$$

Step 3: Divide by 2 on both sides to solve for x alone.

$$30 \div 2 = 2x \div 2$$

Step 4: Solve for x.

$$x = 15 \text{ mL}$$

Step 5: The answer is 15 mL.

Osmolality

Osmolality expresses the number of particles (osmols) in an amount of fluid.

Hint: 1 Osm is equal to 1,000 mOsm.

Our human plasma osmolality is about 280–300 mOsm/L. The osmolality of NS is about 300 mOsm/L and D5W is about 280 mOsm/L. This indicates that our IV fluids and plasma should be isotonic (same number of particles in a cell). If parenteral solutions are not isotonic, the result could irritate veins and cause swelling in the red blood cells. These solutions are called hypertonic solutions. If a parenteral solution has less osmolalities than plasma, this is called hypotonic solutions.

The **milliosmol** numbers are very important for clinicians to determine whether the solution is hyperosmotic or hypoosmotic with regard to biological fluids and membranes of the patient.

$$\text{mOsm/L} = \frac{\text{weight of substance (g/L)}}{\text{molecular weight (g)}} \times \text{number of species} \times 1{,}000$$

Example of calculating millimolar value:

How many milliosmoles are represented in a liter of 0.9% sodium chloride solution?

Note: Osmotic concentration (in terms of milliosmoles) is the total number of particles present in a solution. Assuming a complete dissociation, 1 mmol of sodium chloride (NaCl) represents 2 mOsm of total particles (Na^+ and Cl^-).

Formula weight of NaCl = 58.5
1 mmol of NaCl (58.5 mg) = 2 mOsm
0.9% (w/v) = 0.9 g × 1,000 mg / 1 g = 9,000 mg of NaCl per liter

Step 1: Use the proportion formula to set up an equation as follows:

$$\frac{58.5 \text{ mg}}{9{,}000 \text{ mg}} = \frac{2 \text{ mOsm}}{x \text{ mOsm}}$$

Step 2: Cross multiply.

$$58.5 \times x = 9{,}000 \times 2$$

Step 3: Divide by 58.5 on both sides to solve for x alone.
Step 4: Solve for x.
Step 5: Answer is $x = 307.7$ or 308 mOsm.

Please select the correct answer.

1. If an order is written for 60 mEq KCl po bid, what volume of KCl elixir containing 20 mEq / 15 mL will be required to deliver a *single dose*?
    a. 10 mL
    b. 15 mL
    c. 30 mL
    d. 45 mL

2. A prescription order calls for potassium chloride (KCl) 30 mEq in 1,000 mL normal saline. Calculate the number of milliliters that will give this amount from a 2 mEq/mL vial.
    a. 5 mL
    b. 7.5 mL
    c. 10 mL
    d. 15 mL

3. You have D5W and a vial of NaCl (4 mEq/mL). How many mEq would you need to prepare 500 mL of D5W-NS solution? Hint: 15.4 mEq Na+ in every 100 mL of 0.9NS solution.
    a. 15.4 mEq per liter

  b. 77 mEq per liter
  c. 154 mEq per liter
  d. None of the above

4. What is the concentration in milligram per milliliter of a solution containing 2 mEq of potassium chloride (KCl) per milliliter? Hint: molecular weight of KCl = 74.5, *1 mEq of KCl = 74.5 mg.*
  a. 74.5 mg per mL
  b. 149 mg per mL
  c. 223.5 mg per mL
  d. None of the above

5. How many milliosmoles are in half a liter of a 0.9% sodium chloride?
  a. 15.4 mOsm
  b. 154 mOsm
  c. 307 mOsm
  d. None of the above

Chapter 11

Percentage, Percentage Strength, and Ratio Strength

The term *percent* (%) means "per hundred" or "by the hundred" or "in a hundred."

Example: 50% means 50 per 100 or $^{50}/_{100}$.

Below are the four different ways to express percentage:
1. Convert percent to decimal (move decimal two places to the left and drop the percent sign).
   Ex.: 50% = 0.5
2. Convert decimal to percent (move decimal two places to the right and add the percent sign).
   Ex.: 0.5 = 50%
3. Convert percent to proper fraction (divide by 100 and reduce to lowest term).
   Ex.: 50% = $^{50}/_{100}$ or ½
4. Convert proper fraction to percent (first convert to decimal and multiply by 100).
   Ex.: ¼ = 0.25 = (0.25 × 100) = 25%

A. *Percentage* (%) is the number of parts per 100 parts. It is an expression of the desired amount in a given total volume or total weight (i.e., 1% [w/w] hydrocortisone = 1 g HC in a 100 g ointment). This is an example of weight over weight.

Whenever working on a percentage problem, always convert the problems to a fraction.

There are three different types:

    a. (W/W) = (weight/weight) or solid/solid = number of active ingredient in grams per 100 grams

b. (V/V) = (volume/volume) or liquid/liquid = number of active ingredient in ml per 100 mL
c. (W/V) = weight/volume or solid/liquid) = number of active ingredient in grams per 100 ml

Examples of the discussion above, respectively:

a. Hydrocortisone 1% (w/w) cream is equal to 1 gr of hydrocortisone in 100 g of ointment.
b. The 70% (v/v) isopropyl alcohol is equal to 70 mL of alcohol in 100 mL of water.
c. Dextrose in 5% (w/v) water is equal to 5 g of dextrose in 100 mL of water.

B. **Percentage strength** is a solution that contains solid dissolved in liquid. This is the mathematical expression of the concentration of a solution. By convention, a *percentage strength* is the number of grams of ingredients in 100 ml of product.

1. Set up as a fraction with ratio strength over 100%.
2. Set up as a fraction with known number of parts over unknown parts.
3. Set up proportion equation.
4. Cross multiply, then solve for x.
5. Set up ratio.

Example: What is the ratio strength of 0.005%?

1. $\dfrac{0.005\%}{100}$

2. $\dfrac{1 \text{ part}}{x \text{ parts}}$

3. $\dfrac{0.005\%}{100\,\%} = \dfrac{1 \text{ part}}{x \text{ part}}$

4. $x = 20,000$

5. Set up as ratio = 1:20,000

Find the *ratio strength* for the following:

1. 0.025%

2. 0.001%

3. 0.02%

4. 0.0125%

5. 0.00025%

C. **Ratio strength** is a solution that contains solid dissolved in liquid. This is the mathematical expression of a concentration of a solution. By convention, ratio strength 1:2,000 w/v means 1 g in 2,000 ml. Usually, concentration of a weak solution is expressed as ratio strength.

1. Express ratio strength as fraction.
2. Set up as a fraction with known number of parts over unknown parts.
3. Set up 1 and 2 together to form a proportion equation to solve for x.
4. Cross multiply, then solve for x.

Example: Convert 1:20,000 to a percentage strength. This means that there is 1 gr of active ingredient in a 20,000 ml solution.

1. $\dfrac{1 \text{ part}}{20,000}$

2. $\dfrac{x\%}{100\%}$

3. $\dfrac{1 \text{ part}}{20{,}000 \text{ parts}} = \dfrac{x\%}{100\%}$

4. Cross multiply, then solve for x.
   Answer: $x = 0.005\%$

Find the percentage strength for the following:

1. 1:8,000

2. 1:80,000

3. 1:20,000

4. 1:10,000

5. 1:100,000

Chapter 12

Calculating Dosage

Dosage calculation is very useful for a pharmacy technician when it comes to reading the doctor's prescription. Interpreting prescriptions can be challenging. Physicians use prescription abbreviations (based on Latin words) which tell the pharmacist which drugs to give and how to use that medication. As a pharmacy technician, one will use their math extensively to interpret orders and perform pharmacy calculations and to memorize the abbreviation list. This list can be found on the back of this book.

See the formula below:

$$\frac{\text{Total medication}}{\text{Size of one dose}} = \text{Number of doses}$$

This formula can be rearranged in the following two ways:

$$\frac{\text{Size of one dose}}{\text{Number of doses}} = \text{Total medication}$$

or

$$\frac{\text{Number of doses}}{\text{Size of one dose}} = \text{Total medication}$$

A. *Calculating total medication*

Example: How many milliliters would you need to prepare a prescription if the doctor ordered 1 teaspoon on the first day then ½ teaspoonful daily for four days?

Note: First, calculate the total number of doses the patient needs to receive. Then multiply this number by the dose.

$$\text{Total medication} = \frac{\text{Number of doses}}{\text{Size of one dose}}$$

$$\begin{aligned}
1 \text{ teaspoon} = 5 \text{ mL}; \tfrac{1}{2} \text{ tsp} &= 2.5 \text{ mL} \\
5 \text{ mL} + (2.5 \text{ mL} \times 4 \text{ days}) &= x \\
5 \text{ mL} + 10 \text{ mL} &= x \\
15 \text{ mL} &= x
\end{aligned}$$

B. *Calculating dose size*

Example: If a patient is to receive a total of 600 mg of theophylline each day and the patient takes one dose every twelve hours, how many milligrams are in each dose?

Note: First, calculate how many times the patient takes the medication in a day. There are twenty-four hours in a day. If the patient takes one dose every twelve hours, he takes one dose two times a day.

$$\frac{\text{Size of one dose}}{\text{Number of doses}} = \text{Total medication}$$

$$x \text{ (size of one dose)} = \frac{600 \text{ mg}}{2 \text{ times a day}}$$

$$x \text{ (size of one dose)} = 300 \text{ mg}$$

C. *Calculating number of doses*

Example: How many 30 mL doses can be made out of 1 gal?

Note: Calculate the number of doses in a specified amount of medicine.

$$\text{Number of doses} = \frac{\text{Total medication}}{\text{Size of one dose}}$$

Note: 1 gal = 4,000 mL

4,000 mL ÷ 30 mL doses = number of doses

Answer: 133.33, which is ~ 134 doses

Practice Questions

1. If the dose of a drug is 55 mcg, how many doses are contained in 0.055 g?

2. If a preparation contains 5 g of a drug in 500 mL, how many grams are contained in a 2 tbsp dose?

3. A 10 kg child receives 100 mg q8h of amoxicillin. The usual dosage is 50 mg/kg per day divided into three doses. How many milligram would this child receive in a day based from the recommendation of 50 mg/kg/day?

4. How many 10 mL doses can be made out of 1 pt?

5. How many milliliters of ampicillin do you have to dispense if the patient needs to take 2 tsp four times a day for ten days?

6. A liquid medicine contains 0.025 mg/ml of a substance. How many milligram of the substance will 1.5 L contain?

7. How many teaspoonfuls would be prescribed in each dose of an elixir if 6 fl oz contained twenty doses?

8. How many drops would be prescribed in each dose of a liquid medicine if 12 mL contained sixty doses? Note that a dropper calibrates 30 gtts per mL.

9. How many milligrams of a drug substance are required to make 100 mL of a solution with each teaspoonful of which contains 5 mg of the drug substance?

10. A drug concentration is 100 mg / 2.5 mL. If a dose of 100 mg is administered QID, the total daily dose would be?
    a. 2.5 mL containing 400 mg
    b. 5 mL containing 0.4 g
    c. 10 mL containing 0.4 g
    d. 10 mL containing 40 g

Chapter 13

Calculating Day Supply

Calculating day supply is very important, especially when billing to the third-party health care for reimbursement. If inaccurately calculated, the day supply can cause the beneficiary to receive the incorrect amount of medication and may even result in rejections or possibly raise audit red flags.

To calculate the day supply, the pharmacist or technician should divide the given or calculated quantity by the number of dose per day. For instance, to calculate the day supply for inhalers, first calculate the total number of actuations to be dispensed by multiplying the number of actuations per inhaler by the number of inhalers to be dispensed. Then divide the total number of actuations or doses to be dispensed by the number of doses required daily.

Calculating the day supply is not always easy. It is recommended to follow the standard billing units for consistency per insurance agencies, such as milliliter, grams, 1 pump equals to 1 gram or 1 gram per unit dose, and so forth.

Example: Proventil HFA inhaler contains 200 metered inhalations. If a patient inhaled two puffs orally for four to six hours, not to exceed twelve inhalations per twenty-four hours, how many days will this Proventil HFA inhaler last?

1. Calculate the total actuations in this one Proventil HFA inhaler.
   Answer: Two hundred actuations.

2. How many inhalations will be used in a day or in a twenty-four-hour period?
   Answer: Twelve inhalations.

3. Two hundred total actuations divided by twelve inhalations per day is equal to a day supply.
   Answer: 16.67 days or 17 days' supply.

Practice Questions

1. How many days' supply will two boxes of Climara patch 0.1 mg last when the patient applies one patch once a week? Note that the box comes with four patches.

2. The doctor writes a prescription for Estraderm 0.05 mg patch / twenty-four patches with the direction to apply one patch BIW. How many days' supply will the prescription last?

3. A prescription is written for Medrol Dosepak (methylprednisolone) 4 mg tablet, containing twenty-one tablets, with the instruction to take six tablets on the first day, then decrease by one tablet until it's gone (6-5-4-3-2-1). How many days' supply will this Dosepak last?

4. How many days' supply will an eye drop of 2.5 mL last if a patient instills 1 gtt ou QHS?
Note: 1 ml delivers 20 drops.

5. If a doctor writes a prescription for 240 g of calcipotriene 0.005% cream with the instruction of applying one to two grams topically to affected area three to four times daily, how many days' supply will this tube of medicine last?

6. A bottle of 8-ounces Flurandrenolide 0.05% lotion was prescribed with an instruction of apply 1-3 ml to affected area two to three times daily for itching/eczema.?

7. A prescription is written for Dihydroergotamine mesylate 4 mg/ml vial; SIG: Use 1 spray (0.5 mg) in each nostril. If needed repeat after 15-30 mins for a maximum total of 4 sprays (2 mg) per 24 hour period. The recommendation for a maximum is eight sprays a week. The doctor is written for a quantity of 1 box which contains 8 vials. How many days would 8 vials last the patient?

8. A wound prescription, Mupirocin 2% cream, was prescribed for bacterial infection with an instruction of apply 2-4 grams topically three times daily for a quantity of 300 grams. How many days would this 300 grams last the patient?

9. A bottle of 10 ml insulin Humulin R was prescribed for a diabetic patient to use for his high blood sugar with an instruction of 5 units subcutaneous ACHS. How long would this 1 bottle of insulin last the patient? Note: 1 ml equals 100 units.

10. A doctor wrote a prescription for an arthritis patient, a Diclofenac topical solution with an instruction to apply 2-3 ml three to four times daily to affected area for pain (20 drops = 1ml). How many days does this prescription last the patient if the doctor prescribed 2 bottles, each bottle contains 150 ml?

Chapter 14

Calculating Children's Dosage

There are four different types of formulas to calculate children's dosage. Each of these use different body data. It is either using one of the following: weight as in age or as in years, months, pounds, or age at next birthday. Thus note that children have much difference in weight and tolerance.

When working with children dose, one must be cautiously double check or even triple check to make sure the correct calculation perform.

Children's Doses (Hint: 1 kg = 2.2 lb)

Clark's Rule	$\dfrac{\text{Weight of child}}{150 \text{ lb}}$	× Adult dose	= Dose for child
Young's Rule	$\dfrac{\text{Age of child}}{\text{Age} + 12}$	× Adult dose	= Dose for child
Fried's Rule	$\dfrac{\text{Age of child (month)}}{150}$	× Adult dose	= Dose for child
Cowling's Rule	$\dfrac{\text{Age at next birthday (in years)}}{24}$	× Adult dose	= Dose for child

Practice Questions

1. If the adult dose of a drug is 60 mg, what would be the dose for a child weighing 35 lb? Use *Clark's rule*.

Use the following problem for questions 2 and 3:

A patient who weighs 25 kg receives 200 mg of acyclovir suspension Q8H. The adult dose is 800 mg.

2. What is the dose for a five-year-old child if we use *Young's rule*?

3. What would be the dose using *Clark's rule*?

Use the following problem for questions 4 and 5:

The usual dose of sulfisoxazole suspension for infants over two months of age and children is 60 mg/kg of body weight. Adult dose of sulfisoxazole is 500 mg

4. Use *Fried's rule* to calculate the child's dose if the patient is 5 months old.
5. Use *Cowling's rule* to calculate the child's dose if the patient has a next birthday in three more months he will be 6 years old.

Chapter 15

Dilution Method

Most diluted admixture solutions are usually stocked in the hospital pharmacy. These dilution solutions are usually prepared from a stock solution. To prepare a solution of the desired concentration, one must calculate the volume of stock solution by mixing it with either diluents or another lower concentration to prepare the final concentration. For instance, if the mixture of a given percentage is diluted to twice its original quantity, then its strength will be reduced by one-half. If a mixture is concentrated by evaporation to one-half its original quantity, then the strength will be doubled.

This is the dilution formula:

(Initial volume × Initial strength) = (Final volume × Final strength)
    (Iv)   ×   (Is)   =   (Fv)   ×   (Fs)

Hint: Anytime you see the words *of*, *times*, and *multiplied by*, it signals multiplication.

Initial volume (Iv) = initial volume (the volume with which you started out)
Initial strength (Is) = initial strength (the concentration with which you started out)
Final volume (Fv) = the final volume with which you want to end up
Final strength (Fs) = the final strength or concentration with which you want to end up

Remember, initial volume is always less than the final volume because you've added water. The final strength is less than the initial strength because you've diluted it with water.

Example: You have a 70% (v/v) isopropyl alcohol stock solution available. You need to prepare 300 ml of 10% (v/v) isopropyl alcohol.

How many milliliters of the stock solution do you need to make this preparation?

Dilution formula = Initial volume × Initial strength = Final volume × Final strength

$$x \times 70\% = 300 \text{ ml} \times 10\%$$
$$70x = 3000 \text{ ml}$$
$$\frac{70x}{70} = \frac{3{,}000}{70}$$
$$x = 42.85 \text{ mL}$$

Practice Problems

1. How many milliliters of a 40% stock solution can be made from 2 L of a 25% solution?

2. If a gallon of 20% solution is to be evaporated so that the solution will have a strength of 45%, what will its volume be in milliliters?

3. How many milliliters of a 2% stock solution of ephedrine sulfate should be used in compounding 30 mL of 0.25% ephedrine sulfate solution?

4. How many milliliters of water should be added to 100 mL of a 1:200 solution of benzalkonium chloride to make a 1:2,500 solution?

5. How many milliliters of 90% alcohol and how much water should be added to a liter of a 12% solution?

6. What is the percentage of alcohol in a cough mixture containing half a liter of terpin hydrate elixir and 100 mL of chloroform spirit? Terpin hydrate elixir contains 40% alcohol, while chloroform spirit contains 90% alcohol.

7. How many grams of a 20% trituration of atropine sulfate should be used in preparing 350 mL of a solution of atropine sulfate which is to contain $\frac{1}{400}$ g of atropine per 5 mL?

8. How much silver nitrate should be used in preparing 30 mL of a solution such that its 5 mL diluted to 500 mL will yield a 1:1,000 solution?

9. How much water should be added to 1,375 mL of 81% alcohol to prepare 45% alcohol?

10. What volume of 2.5% sodium hypochlorite is required to prepare 1 L of 0.1% sodium hypochlorite–disinfecting solution?

Chapter 16

Pharmacy Alligations

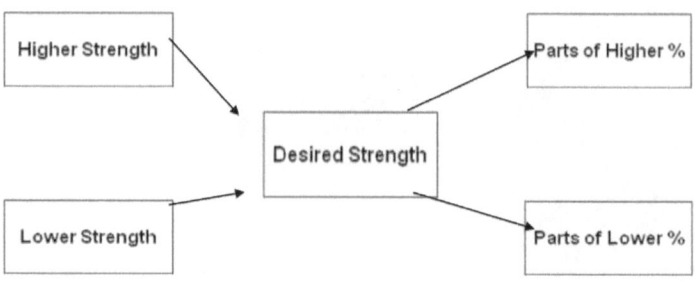

What is *alligation aliquot*?

It is a method used to calculate the desired concentration of a solution by mixing together three or more different percentage concentrations of the same active ingredient together. Thus, the strength of the final product will fall in between the strengths of the original product. This calculation is used to determine the number of parts for each concentration.

- A. Set up a tic-tac-toe and fill in the slot.
- B. Set up as proportion equation and solve for x part for each strength.
- C. Set up as proportion equation and solve for x mL of each part.

Note: They must have the same units and no negative number.

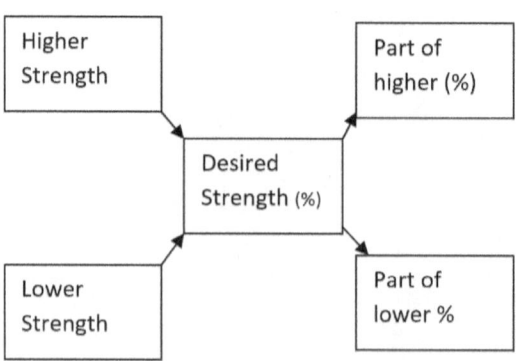

I. *Single alligation*

To obtain 500 mL of 55% dextrose solution, how many milliliters of 75% and 35% solutions will you need?

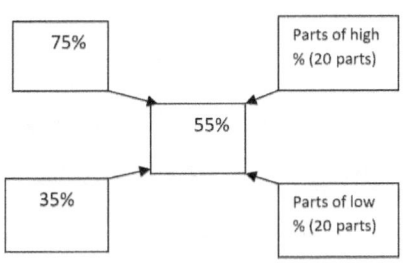

Below are the steps in solving alligation problems:

1. Place the total percentage of strength on the appropriate block.

2. Determine the parts for each percentage.

3. Keep in mind that the desired percentage is given—i.e., 55% dextrose of 500 mL has total parts (40 parts).

4. Determine the volume (mL) for each part by using proportion.

Determine the volume (ml) for each part by using proportion, or determine how many milliliter per each part.

500 mL divided by 40 parts = 12.5 mL = 1 part

a. 20 parts of 75% = 20 parts × 12.5mL/part

x = 250 mL

b. 20 parts of 35% = 20 parts × 12.5mL/part

x = 250 mL

Add the sum of both volumes together. It should be equal to 500 mL

Note: Add the sum of both volumes. It should equal to the total volume.
250 mL + 250 mL = 500 mL

II. *Double alligation*

In what proportion should amino acid of 30%, 15%, and 5% strength be mixed to make a liter of 20% amino acid solution? How much milliliters of each solution of 30%, 15%, and 5%, respectively?

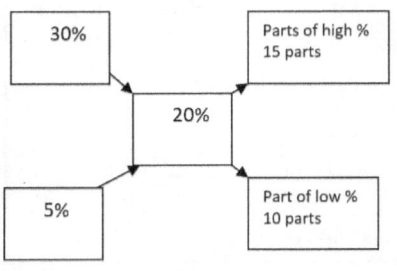 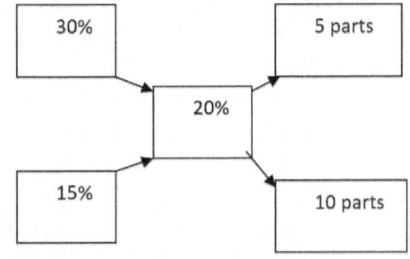

69

Summary of all parts

15 parts of 30%
5 parts of 30%
10 parts of 15%
<u>10 parts of 5%</u>
40 parts in total

Below are the steps in solving alligation problems:

1. Place percentage strength on the appropriate block.

2. Determine the parts for each percentage.

3. Keep in mind that the desired percentage is given—i.e., 20% amino acid of 1000 mL has total parts (40 parts).

4. Add all parts of the concentration together.

5. Determine the volume (mL) for each part by using proportion.

Determine the volume (mL) for each part by using proportion.

Take a given volume of 1000 ml divided by the total parts (40 parts). It is equal to 25 ml. Thus, each part will deliver 25 milliliters.

15 parts of amino acid (AA) 30% × 25 mL = 375 mL
10 parts of 5% of AA × 25 mL = 250 mL
5 parts of 30% of AA × 25 mL = 125 mL
<u>10 parts of 15% of AA × 25 mL = 250 mL</u>
40 parts in total   × 25 mL   = 1000 mL

Practice Questions

1. To obtain a liter of 12.5% amino acid, how many milliliters of 15% amino acid and 10% amino acid will you need?

2. To process a prescription order for a 13% dextrose solution, in what ratio will the pharmacy technician mix the stock solutions of 20% dextrose and 5% dextrose solutions?

3. The pharmacy has a 10% ointment and a 1% ointment, and you are asked to make a 2.5% ointment of 45 g. What parts of each strength will be used? Give the final weight for each needed for the prescription.

4. How many milliliter of 70% alcohol and 40% alcohol should be mixed to prepare 240 mL of 60% alcohol?

5. Aminosyn is an amino acid often used in TPN orders to provide protein for cellular repair and growth. A physician writes an order for 2.5% 500 mL aminosyn. You have aminosyn 8.5% 500 ml. How are you going to prepare this order using a sterile evacuated container?

6. How many grams of 3% Digel should be mixed with 200 grams of 0.5% Digel to make a 1% Digel?

7. We wish to dilute an ointment containing 10% of sulfur with petrolatum to make 100 grams of an ointment containing 5% sulfur. How many grams of 10% sulfur ointment and how many grams of petrolatum will be necessary to make the dilution?

8. How many grams of 2.5% compound "HC" cream should be mixed with 150 grams of 0.375% compound "HC" cream to make a 0.5% cream?

9. You receive an order for 50 grams of 0.25% Hydrocortisone cream to use in infant. You have available 1% Hydrocortisone cream and cold cream that can be mixed with the Hydrocortisone. How many grams of the cold cream will be needed to fill the order?

10. To process a prescription order for a 23% dextrose solution, in what ratio will the pharmacy technician mix the stock solutions of 70% dextrose and 10% dextrose solutions?

Chapter 17

Flow Rate Calculation

The calculation of flow rate is essential to ensure that the patients are getting the amount of fluid needed to prevent dehydration or the amount of medication the doctor prescribed for the patient to receive over a period of time.

Flow rate is the total amount of volume run over a specific amount of time (volume [mL] / time [minute or hour]).

    a. It is often expressed in these units:
       • mL/hr   • mL/min   • gtt/hr   • gtt/min
    b. An important part is how you set up the equation using *cancellation method.*
    c. Always pay attention to the *unit* for which the question is looking.

Note: One hour is equal to sixty minutes. This is commonly used in these types of problem.

Calculate flow rate and drip rate (for tubing).
Always express in mL per minute (mL/min) or gtts per minute (gtt/min).

    macrodrip   =   1 mL   =   10 gtts
    microdrip   =   1 mL   =   60 gtts

The canceling method is very useful when working with flow rate problems by drawing a horizontal straight line from the left to the right. Always start with the unit the question is asking for, and cancel out all the units that look alike. Leave only the remaining units that they ask for. All the numerators multiply together and will be divided by all the denominators to obtain your answer.

Practice Questions

1. A solution is to be administered by IV infusion at a rate of 140 mL/h. How many gtt/min. should be infused if 1 mL = 25 gtts?

2. A patient is to receive 1,000 mL of IV solution over ten hours. What is the rate of infusion (gtt/min) that should be utilized if 1 mL = 20 gtts?

3. An order is written for 20 g of lidocaine in 500 mL of D5W to infuse at 100 mg/hr. What is the rate of infusion in mL/hr?

4. An order is written for 25,000 units of heparin in 250 mL of 0.45NS. The doctor instructs to infuse 25 mL/hr. How many units of heparin will the patient receive in a twelve-hour period?

5. An IV drip provides 20 gtts/mL. The physician orders a 100 mL bag of dextrose to be administered at a flow rate of 10 gtts/min. How long will it take to administer the entire bag?

6. Given LR 1 L with 10,000 units of heparin at 1,200 unit/hr, how long would it take for the patient to receive 120 mL?

7. A solution is to be administered by IV solution at a rate of 140 mL/hr. How many gtt/min should be infused if 1 mL = 25 drops?

8. A patient is to receive 1,000 mL of IV solution over twelve hours. What is the rate of infusion (gtt/min) that should be utilized if 1 mL = 16 gtts?

9. An IV drip provides 12 gtts/mL. The physician orders a 250 mL bag of dextrose to be administered at a flow rate of 10 gtts/min. How long will it take to administer the entire bag?

10. If a continuous renal replacement therapy (CRRT) of a 3 L bag is infused over two hours each bag, what is the rate of infusion in mL/hr?

Chapter 18

Commercial Calculations and Terminology

Pharmacy technicians should be familiar with the following terminology and have a basic understanding the concepts of business calculations when working in retail pharmacy.

Cost — The cost of a drug (acquisition cost)

Markup — The difference between the cost and its selling price. In other words, it's our profit.

Selling price — The total cost of a drug plus markup or gross profit

Gross profit — The difference between the selling price and the cost of an item

Percent markup — A percentage of the cost

Overhead — The expenses of the pharmacy in conducting business such as salaries, rent, utilities, freight costs, interest, taxes, and others

Inventory — An itemized statement of all the drugs or merchandise on hand

Turnover — The number of times a drug or merchandise is sold in a given length of time

Gross sales — The amount of money received for goods sold within a given length of time

AWP — (average wholesale price) The range of costs of a medication determined by a manufacturer to set prices at different pharmacies

Formulas:

$$\text{Selling price} = \text{Cost} + \text{Markup}$$

$$\text{Markup} = \text{Percentage markup} \times \text{cost}$$

$$\text{Percentage markup} = (\text{Markup} \div \text{Cost}) \times 100$$

$$\text{Net profit} = \text{Selling price} - (\text{Cost} + \text{Overhead})$$

Practice questions

1. The cost of a Z-Pak, an antibiotic, is $34.50, and the selling price is $59.69. What is the percentage of the markup and its amount?

2. You have a prescription for a 45 g Differin 0.3% gel. This costs you $90. You want to use a 50% markup on the cost. What is the retail price to the customer?

3. Mr. Smith has a written prescription for a 10 mg Lipitor (a brand drug that costs $110). He is on Aetna insurance. It requires a $50 deductible for each member of the family. Once the deductible has met, he will pay $20 for the brand and $10 for generic. However, Mr. Smith has not met his deductible yet for the new year. What is his total copayment?

4. A prescription for thirty capsules of amoxicillin 250 mg has a usual and customary price of $8.49. The acquisition cost of amoxicillin 250 mg #30 is $2.02. What is the gross profit?

5. An insulin Humalog U-100 contains 100 units of insulin per milliliter. The AWP for one 10 mL vial costs $145.00. The acquisition cost to the pharmacy for a 10 mL vial is $98.50. The usual and customary price for one bottle of Humalog at that pharmacy is $89.25. If the pharmacy has an agreement with the third-party plan for reimbursement of 80% AWP or 100% U&C (whichever is less) plus a $5.50 dispensing fee, what will be the total amount of the third-party claim?

    Use the following information to answer question #6, #7, #8, and #9
    Markup = 20% for AWP less than $100
    Markup = $7.50 for AWP $100 or more
    Dispensing fee = $5 per prescription

Compounding fee = $50 per hour
Senior citizen discount = 10%

Dispense the following compounded prescription:
Aquaphor ointment 30 g, AWP $2.50
Cholestyramine powd 4 g, AWP $3.00
Hydrocortisone 1% 30 g, AWP $4.50
Compounding time = 15 min.

6. What is the selling price?
7. What is the selling price for a senior citizen?
8. What is the gross profit?
9. What is the net profit?

Appendix A

Patterned Plan of Attack for Questions

How Do You Solve Word Problems?

There are two steps involved in solving math word problems:
1. Translate the wording into a numeric equation that combines smaller expressions.
2. Solve the equation.

Word problems are often a series of expressions that fit into an equation. An *equation* is a combination of math expressions.

Strongly recommended tips in solving word problems:
1. Read the problem entirely to get the feel of the whole problem and identify what the problem is.
2. List all the given information and identify all the variables. Be sure to write the units of measurement with the variables (i.e., gallons, dollars, milligrams, grams, etc.).
3. Define what answer you would need as well as its unit of measure.
4. Work in an organized manner. Stay in focus and keep in mind what the problem is. If it is necessary, draw and label all graphs and pictures clearly.
5. Look for the key words. They are as follows: *of*, *times*, *multiplied by* (which means multiplication), *per*, *a*, *out of*, *ratio of*, *over*, *percent* (divide by 100 and which means division), *single dose* (which means one dose given to patient), *daily dose* (which means total doses given in one day or twenty-four hours), and *diluted to* (which means adding water [note: water always has 0%]). For example, *per* means "divided by" as in "I drove 90 m on 3 gal of gas, so I got 30 m per gal or 30 m/gal." Here's another example: *a* means "divided by," as in "When I tanked up, I paid $3.90 for 3 gal, so the gas was $1.30 a gal or $1.30/gal."

Appendix B

Patterned Plan of Attack for Calculations

Review of Basic Mathematics Used in Pharmacy

I. *Temperature conversion*

$$°F = \frac{(9 \times C)}{5} + 32 \qquad °C = \frac{5 \times (F - 32)}{9}$$

II. *Roman numerals*

ss	=	½
I	=	1
V	=	5
X	=	10
L	=	50
C	=	100
D	=	500
M	=	1,000

III. *Calculating Drug Enforcement Agency (DEA) number*

1. Add the odd numbers (1, 3, and 5): $1 + 3 + 5 = 9$.

2. Add the even numbers (2, 4, and 6): $2 + 4 + 6 = 12 \times 2 = (24)$.

3. Add the sum of both steps together ($9 + 24 = 33$).

4. The second digit of the sum is the last digit of the DEA number.

Answer: AB 1234563

IV. *Metric system*

mcg	mg	cg	dg	gm	dg	hg	kg	Mg
micro	milli	centi	deci	gram	deka	hecto	kilo	mega
0.000001	0.001	0.01	0.1	1	10	100	1,000	1,000,000

V. *Pharmacy conversion (usually in sig part of prescription)*

Volume: 1 milliliter (mL) = 16 minim (m) (15 drops [gtts])

   1 teaspoon (tsp) = 5 mL
   1 tablespoon (tbsp) = 15 mL
   1 ounce (oz) = 30 mL
   1 pint (pt) = 480 mL
   1 quart (qt) = 2 pint (960 mL)
   1 liter (L) = 1,000 mL or 34 fl oz (1.1 qt)
   1 gallon (Gal) = 4,000 mL (4 quarts = 8 pt)

Weight: 1 grain (gr) = 65 mg
   1 ounce (oz) = 30 g (480 g)
   1 pound (lb) = 454 g
   1 kilogram (kg) = 2.2 lb

VI. *Prescription calculation*

Formula 1   Total medication = $\dfrac{\text{Number of doses}}{\text{Size of one dose}}$

Formula 2   Total medication = $\dfrac{\text{Doses per day} \times \text{number of days}}{\text{Size of one dose}}$

VII. *Children's doses (Hint: 1 kg = 2.2 lb)*

Clark's rule: $\dfrac{\text{Weight of child}}{150 \text{ lb}} \times \text{Adult dose} = \text{Dose for child}$

Young's rule: $\dfrac{\text{Age of child}}{\text{Age} + 12} \times \text{Adult dose} = \text{Dose for child}$

Fried's Rule: $\dfrac{\text{Age of child (month)}}{150} \times \text{Adult dose} = \text{Dose for child}$

Cowling's Rule: $\dfrac{\text{Age at next birthday (in years)}}{24} \times \text{Adult dose} = \text{Dose for child}$

VIII. *Dilution*

Final volume × Final strength = Initial volume × Initial strength

IX. *Alligation*

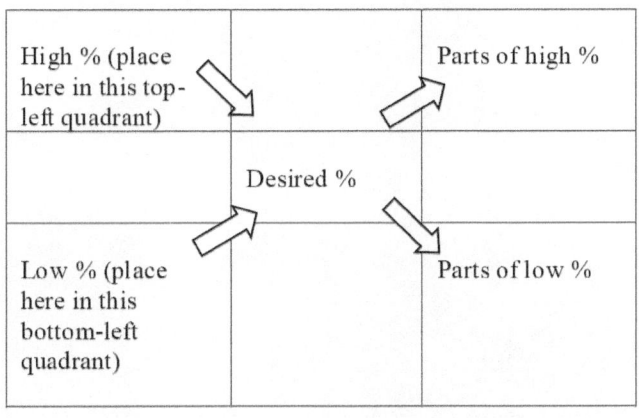

X. *Calculating flow rate and drip rate (for tubing)*
Always express in milliliter per minute (mL/min) or drops (gtts) per min (gtt/min) Recommended use is the cancelation method.

It is often expressed in these units:
- mL/hr • mL/min • gtt/hr • gtt/min

  macrodrip = 1 mL = 10 gtts
  microdrip = 1 mL = 60 gtts

XI. *Commercial calculations*

  Selling price   =   Cost + Markup

  Markup   =   Percentage markup × Cost

  Percentage markup   =   (Markup ÷ Cost) × 100

  Net profit   =   Selling price − (Cost + Overhead)

Appendix C

Common Pharmacy Abbreviations

Application	Time	Application	Areas
QD	every day	AD	right ear
BID	twice daily	AS	left ear
TID	three times daily	AU	both ears
QID	four times daily	Aff ear	affected ear(s)
5XD	five times daily	OD	right eye
QOD	every other day	OS	left eye
Q1H	every 1 hour	OU	both eyes
Q4H	every 1 hour	Aff eye	affected eye(s)
Q4-6H	every 4–6 hours	AA	affected area(s)
Q12H	every 12 hours	BSA	body surface area
Q24H	every 24 hours	SL	under the tongue, sublingual
Q Wk	every week	SC, SQ	subcutaneous, under the skin
BIW	twice a week	Sup, supp.	Suppository
QMonth	every month	SR	suppository rectally
HS	at bedtime	SV	suppository vaginally
AC	before meals	Vag	Vaginally
PC	after meals		

Appendix D

Common Medical Abbreviations

AA, aa	of each
Ad lib	at pleasure
ADR	adverse drug reaction
AM	morning
Amp	ampoule
ANS	autonomic nervous system
APAP	acetaminophen
Aq, aqua	water
Aq dist	distilled water
ASA	aspirin
AWP	average wholesale price
BC	birth control
BE	barium enema
BM	bowel movement
BP	blood pressure
BUN	blood urea nitrogen
C	with
Carb	carbohydrate
Cath	catheter
CC	cubic centimeter
CCU	critical care unit
CHF	congestive heart failure
Cmp.	compound
Conc.	concentration
CVA	cerebral vascular accident
D5W	dextrose 5% in water

DAW	dispense as written
DC	discontinue
DEA	Drug Enforcement Administration
Diag, DX	diagnosis
Disp.	dispense
DS	double strength
DUR	drug utilization (usage) review
ECG	electrocardiogram
EEG	electroencephalogram
El, elix	elixir
Ex aq.	in water
EtOH	ethanol, alcohol
Ext.	extract, external
FBS	fasting blood sugar
Fl, fld	fluid
Gm, g	gram
Gl	gastrointestinal
Gr	grain
Gtt	drop(s)
GU	genitourinary
H	hypodermic
Hr	hour
HA	hyperalimentation, headache
HC	hydrocortisone
HDL	high-density lipoprotein
Hgb	hemoglobin
HIV	human immunodeficiency virus
HMO	health maintenance organization
HR	heart rate

Hx	history
HS	Bedtime
ICU	intensive care unit
IM	intramuscular
INH	isoniazid
INR	international normalized ratio
IV	intravenous
IVP	intravenous push, intravenous pyelogram
Kg	kilogram
Lb	pound
LCD	coal tar solution (liquor carbonis detergens)
LDL	low density lipoprotein
LOC	laxative of choice
M	mix
MAC	maximum allowable cost
Mcg	microgram
MDI	metered dose inhaler
mEq	milliequivalent
m. ft.	mix and make
Mg	milligram
MI	myocardial infarction
Mixt	mixture
ML	milliliter
MM	millimeter
MOM	milk of magnesia
MR	may repeat
MS	morphine sulfate
MVI	multiple vitamin infusion

NandV	nausea and vomiting
NMT	no more than
Non rep, NR	do not repeat
Noc.	night (nocturnal)
NPO	nothing by mouth
NS	normal saline
NSAID	nonsteroidal anti-inflammatory drugs
NTG	nitroglycerin
Oint	ointment
OJ	orange juice
O	pint
OTC	over-the-counter drug, nonprescription
Oz	ounce
PCN	penicillin
Ped	pediatric
PEFR	peak expiratory flow rate, peak flow
PM	afternoon, evening
PO	by mouth, orally
Post	after
Post op	after surgery
Postpartum	after delivery
PPO	preferred provider organization
PPI	patient package insert
Pre op	before surgery
PRN	as needed
PT	prothrombin time
Pulv	powder
Q	each, every
R	right

RBC	red blood cell
R. L., R/L	ringer's lactate
Rx	prescription
S	without
Sat	saturated
Scr	serum creatinine
Sig	label, write on label
SOB	shortness of breath
Sol, soln	solution
SOS	may repeat if necessary
ss	½ (one-half)
SSKI	saturated solution of potassium iodide
STAT	now, immediately
Surg.	surgery
Susp.	suspension
SWI, SWFI	sterile water, sterile water for injection
Sx	symptoms
T	temperature
Tal.	such
Tal Dos.	such dose
Tbsp	tablespoon
TC	total serum cholesterol
TCN	tetracycline
TCT	total clotting time
TPA	tissue plasminogen activator
TPN	total parenteral nutrition
Tinct.	tincture
Top.	topically
Tsp	teaspoon
Ung.	ointment

Ud, ut dict.	as directed
URI	upper respiratory infection
UTI	urinary tract infection
w, wk	weekly

Answers

Addition	Division	Temperature (°F)	Roman Number
1. 71	1. 7.2	1. 89.6°F	1. XIX
2. 114	2. 8 3/7	2. 77°F	2. XXXIV
3. 772	3. 10 ½	3. 57.2°F	3. XLIX
4. 1,040 ¾	4. 7 29/50	4. 48.2°F	4. CXIV
5. 3,992.59	5. 11 11/50	5. 26.6°F	5. CCXLI
6. 999.006	6. 39 45/50	6. 114.8°F	6. DLXXIX
7. 4.922	7. 8 63/100	7. 136.4°F	7. DCLXXXI
8. 624.724	8. 4 43/50	8. 168.8°F	8. CMLXXVIII
9. 11,458.31	9. 0.622	9. 209.5°F	9. MXXI
10. 66,741.7847	10. 4.16	10. 249.8°F	10. VCCCLXIX

Subtraction	Volume	Temperature (°C)	DEA Number
1. 62	1. 210 mL	1. 40°C	1. C
2. 102	2. 18 teaspoons	2. 33.3°C	2. C
3. 292	3. 2,000 mL	3. 24.4°C	3. a. 6, b. 2
4. 362 ½	4. 134	4. 0°C	
5. 2,435.036	5. 35	5. -12.2°C	Fraction
6. 2,636.005	6. 44 pints	6. 13.3°C	1. ¾
7. 7,761.65	7. 59 glasses	7. 25.6°C	2. 1 7/12
8. 1,604.02	8. 11 liters	8. 37°C	3. 5/16
9. 2,009.2	9. 175 gtts	9. 43.3°C	4. ½
10. 4,774.34	10. 30 doses	10. D	5. 3/16
			6. 3/8
			7. 1/16
			8. 5/12
			9. 2
			10. 9

Multiplication	Weight	Arabic Number	Decimals
1. 33,439	1. 10 doses	1. 94	1. 438.26
2. 111,452	2. 12.27 kg	2. 758	2. 690.41
3. 6,708	3. 10,000 doses	3. 493	3. 4.591
4. 159,318	4. 140 g	4. 1998	4. 2.02
5. 645,498	5. 2.08 oz	5. 1991	5. 14.593
6. 1,156,307.29	6. 160.6 lb	6. 2005	6. 312.29
7. 3,593,517	7. 455 mg	7. 2023	7. 3.48
8. 10,187,884	8. 9 gr	8. 2137	8. 2.322
9. 10,264,211	9. 50 mg	9. 3785	9. 50
10. 2,441,810.9375	10. 1,800 mg	10. 1084	10. 4.21

Ratio and Proportion
1. 48 tsp
2. 400 tablets
3. 8.4 mg
4. 725 mg
5. 10 mL
6. 1 mL
7. 0.35 mL
8. 600 drops
9. 10 gr
10. 500 mg / 5 mL

Chapter 13
Calculating Days Supply
1. 56 days
2. 84 days
3. 6 days
4. 25 days
5. 30 days
6. 27 days
7. 56 days
8. 25 days
9. 50 days
10. 25 days

Milliequivalents
1. d
2. d
3. b
4. b
5. b

Chapter 14
Children's Dosage
1. 14 mg
2. 235 mg
3. 293 mg
4. 16.7 mg
5. 125 mg

Ratio Strength
1. 1:4,000
2. 1:100,000
3. 1:5,000
4. 1:8,000
5. 1:400,000

Percentage Strength
1. 0.0125%
2. 0.00125%
3. 0.005%
4. 0.01%
5. 0.001%

Chapter 12
Calculating Dosage
1. 1000 doses
2. 0.3 gm or 300 mg
3. 500 mg/day
4. If 480ml/pint, 48 doses
5. 400 ml
6. 375 mg
7. 36 doses
8. 12 ml has 60 doses=360 gtts/60 doses= 6 gtts/dose
9. 100 mg
10. (C) 10 ml contains 0.4 gm

Chapter 15
Dilution Method
1. 1250 ml
2. 1682 ml
3. 3.75 ml
4. 1250 ml
5. 133.3 ml
6. 34.8%
7. 21.875g
8. 0.03g
9. 2475 ml
10. 40 ml

Chapter 16
Alligations
1. 500 ml of 15% and 500 ml of 10%
2. 8/15 and 7/15
3. 7.5 g of 1.5 parts of 10%
37.5g of 7.5 parts of 1%
4. 160 ml of 70% and 80 ml of 40%
5. 147 ml of 8.5% and 353 ml of water
6. 40 g of Digel 3% and 160 gm of 0.5% Digel
7. 50 g of 10% and 50 g of petrolatum

8. 8.8 g of 2.5% and 141.2g of 0.375%
9. 12.5 g of 1% and 37.5 gm of cold cream
10. 217 ml of 70% and 783 ml of 10%

Chapter 17
Flow Rates
1. ~58 gtt/min
2. ~33 gtt/min
3. 2.5 ml/hr

4. 30,000 units
5. 200 min or 3 ⅓ hrs
6. 1 hr
7. 24,000 ml or 8 bags of 3 Liters

8. 22.2 gtt/min
9. 300 minutes or 5 hours

10. 1500 ml/hr

Chapter 18
Commercial
1. 42.20%
2. $135
3. $70
4. $6.47
5. $95.00
6. $29.50
7. $26.55
8. $19.50

References

DiPiro, Joseph T. *Clinical Pharmacokinetics and Pharmacodynamics, Pharmacotherapy.* 6th ed. 1999.

Drug Topics. "2009 Top 200 Branded Drugs by Retail Dollars." 2010.

"2009 Top 200 Generic Drugs by Retail Dollars." 2010.

Engel, Kathleen. *Physician Desk Reference.* 64th ed. 2010.

Gahart, B. L. and A. R. Nazareno. *Intravenous Medications.* 25th ed. 2009.

Kastrup, Erwin K., et al. *Drug Facts and Comparisons.* 2010.

Lacy, Charles F., et al. *Lexi-com's Drug Reference Handbook.* 18th ed. 2009–2010.

Michigan Pharmacists Association. *Pharmacy Certified Technician Training Manual.* 1997.

Pharmacist's Letter. *Natural Medicines Comprehensive Database.* http://naturaldatabase.therapeuticresearch.com. Accessed on December 6, 2018.

Schafermeyer, K., and E. Hobson. *The Community Retail Pharmacy Technician Manual.* 1997.

Schneekluth, Gregory. *USP Chapter 797 Clean Room Application.* 2009.

Thomas, Clayton L. *Taber's Cyclopedic Medical Dictionary.* 1993.

Tierney, Lawrence M., Jr., et al. *Antidotes, Current Medical Diagnosis & Treatment.* 35th ed. 2009. 1920.

Trissel, Lawrence A. *Handbook on Injectable Drugs.* 15th ed. 2009.

Troy, David B. *Remington: The Science and Practice of Pharmacy.* 2006.

US Food and Drug Administration. www.fda.gov. Accessed on December 20th, 2018.

Ward, Harold. *Herbal Manual: The Medicinal, Toilet, Culinary and Other Uses of 130 of the Most Commonly Used Herbs.* 1967.

Wilroy, L. J., D. Garcia, and N. T. P. Parks. *National Intravenous Training Manual for Pharmacy Technicians.* 2009.

Index

A

addition, 14
  decimals, 14, 38
  fractions, 14, 38
  whole numbers or integers, 14
alligation
  double, 69
  single, 69
alligation aliquot, 68
  calculation of, 68
average wholesale price (AWP), 76

C

canceling method, 73
Celsius, 30
  conversion formula, 30, 81
certified pharmacy technicians (CPhT), 7, 9
children's dosage, 62, 83
  Clark's rule, 62, 83
  Cowling's rule, 62
  Fried's rule, 62
  Young's rule, 62, 83
commercial calculations, formulas for, 76, 84
concentration, osmotic, 46
cost, 76

D

day supply, 7, 58–59
  calculation of, 58
decimals
  addition of, 14, 38
  division of, 23, 39
  multiplication of, 20, 39
  subtraction of, 17, 38
denominators, 14–15, 18, 38, 73

dilution, 64–65, 71, 83
  final strength (Fs), 64
  final volume (Fv), 64
  initial strength (Is), 64
  initial volume (Iv), 64
dividend, 23
division, 23
  decimals, 23, 39
  fractions, 23, 38
  whole numbers or integers, 23
divisor, 23
dosage calculation, 53
  calculating dose size, 54
  calculating number of doses, 54
  calculating total medication, 53
  formula, 53
drip rate, calculation of, 73, 84
Drug Enforcement Administration (DEA), 36, 81
  calculating the DEA number, 36, 81
  determining last digit of the DEA number, 36
durable medical equipment (DME), 11

E

electrolyte, 44
extremes, 41

F

Fahrenheit, 30
  conversion formula, 30, 81
flow rate, 73
  calculation of, 73, 84
fractions
  addition of, 14, 38
  division of, 23, 38
  multiplication of, 21, 38
  types of

complex fraction, 38
improper fraction, 38
mixed numbers, 38
proper fraction, 38

G

gross profit, 76
gross sales, 76

I

intravenous (IV), 11, 74–75
inventory, 76
ionic charges, 44
isotonic, 46

L

lowest common denominator (LCD), 14–15, 38

M

markup, 76
math
  basic
    addition, 14
    division, 23
    multiplication, 20
    subtraction, 17
  business, 10
  pharmacy, 7, 10
means, 41
metric system, 25–26, 82
milliequivalents, 44
  abbreviation of, 44
milliosmoles
  calculating millimolar value, 46
  formula, 46
multiplication, 20
  decimals, 20, 39
  fractions, 21, 38
  whole numbers or integers, 20

N

National Certified Pharmacy Board, 7
numerators, 15, 18, 38, 73

O

osmolality, 46
  human plasma, 46
osmols, 46
Overhead, 76, 84
over-the-counter (OTC), 11

P

percent, 49
  decimal to percent, 49
  percent to decimal, 49
  percent to proper fraction, 49
  proper fraction to percent, 49
percentage, 49
  types of
    volume/volume, 50
    weight/volume, 50
    weight/weight, 49
percentage strength, 50
percent markup, 76
pharmaceutical conversions, common, 26
  volume, 26
  weight, 26
pharmacy conversion systems
  apothecary, 26
  avoirdupois, 26
Pharmacy Technician Certification Board (PTCB), 9
pharmacy technicians, 7, 9, 13, 26, 41, 53, 76, 98
  duties of, 9, 11, 13
  tasks not performed by, 13
prescription, calculation of, 82
prescriptions, controlled, 36
proportion, 27, 42

solving proportion problems, 42
solving unknown quantities, 42

R

ratio, 41, 50–51, 71, 79
   extremes, 41
   means, 41
ratio strength, 51
roman numerals, 33, 81
   interpretation of, 33

S

selling price, 76
SIG, 26, 60, 82
solutions
   diluted admixture, 64
   electrolyte, 44
   hypertonic, 46
   hypotonic, 46
   parenteral, 46
   stock, 64
subtraction, 17
   decimals, 17, 38
   fractions, 17, 38
   whole numbers or integers, 17

T

temperatures
   Celsius, 30
   Fahrenheit, 30
turnover, 76

U

unit of measure, 79
US Pharmacopeia, 44

V

variables, 79
volume, 26, 28

W

weight, 26, 29
whole numbers or integers
   addition of, 14
   division of, 23
   multiplication of, 20
   subtraction of, 17
word problems, 79
   tips in solving, 79

www.ingramcontent.com/pod-product-compliance
Lightning Source LLC
Chambersburg PA
CBHW021448210526
45463CB00002B/686